©
Copyright 2022 - All rights reserved.

You may not reproduce, duplicate or send the contents of this book without direct written permission from the author. You cannot apply hereby despite any circumstance blame the publisher or hold him or her to legal responsibility for any reparation, compensations, or monetary forfeiture owing to the information included herein, either in a direct or an indirect way.

Legal Notice: This book has copyright protection. You can use the book for personal purposes. You should not sell, use, alter, distribute, quote, take excerpts, or paraphrase in part or whole the material contained in this book without obtaining the permission of the author first.

Disclaimer Notice: You must take note that the information in this document is for casual reading and entertainment purposes only. We have made every attempt to provide accurate, up-to-date, and reliable information. We do not express or imply guarantees of any kind. The persons who read admit that the writer is not occupied in giving legal, financial, medical, or other advice. We put this book content by sourcing various places.

Please consult a licensed professional before you try any techniques shown in this book. By going through this document, the book lover comes to an an agreement that under no situation is the author accountable for any forfeiture, direct or indirect, which they may incur because of the use of material contained in this document, including, but not limited to, — errors, omissions, or inaccuracies.

WORKOUT
Log Book For Men

Belongs to

Name
_____

Adress
_____
_____

Phone
_____

Start Date
_____
End Date
_____

Goals for Today _____ (M) (T) (W) (T) (F) (S) (S)

Muscle Group Focus _____ Weight _____ Date/Time _____

Stretch ○ Warm-Up _____

Strength Training

Exercise	Set	1	2	3	4	5	6	7
	Reps							
	Weight							
	Reps							
	Weight							
	Reps							
	Weight							
	Reps							
	Weight							
	Reps							
	Weight							
	Reps							
	Weight							
	Reps							
	Weight							
	Reps							
	Weight							

Cardio

Exercise	Calories	Distance	Time

Water intake _____

Cooldown _____

Feeling ☆☆☆☆☆

Notes

Goals for Today _____ Ⓜ Ⓣ Ⓦ Ⓣ Ⓕ Ⓢ Ⓢ

Muscle Group Focus _____ Weight _____ Date/Time _____

Stretch ○ Warm-Up _____

Strength Training

Exercise	Set	1	2	3	4	5	6	7
	Reps							
	Weight							
	Reps							
	Weight							
	Reps							
	Weight							
	Reps							
	Weight							
	Reps							
	Weight							
	Reps							
	Weight							
	Reps							
	Weight							
	Reps							
	Weight							

Cardio

Exercise	Calories	Distance	Time

Water intake _____

Cooldown _____

Feeling ☆☆☆☆☆

Notes

Goals for Today _____ (M) (T) (W) (T) (F) (S) (S)

Muscle Group Focus _____ Weight _____ Date/Time _____

Stretch ○ Warm-Up _____

Strength Training

Exercise	Set	1	2	3	4	5	6	7
	Reps							
	Weight							
	Reps							
	Weight							
	Reps							
	Weight							
	Reps							
	Weight							
	Reps							
	Weight							
	Reps							
	Weight							
	Reps							
	Weight							
	Reps							
	Weight							

Cardio

Exercise	Calories	Distance	Time
_____			
_____			
_____			

Water intake _____

Cooldown _____

Feeling ☆☆☆☆☆

Notes

Goals for Today _____ Ⓜ Ⓣ Ⓦ Ⓣ Ⓕ Ⓢ Ⓢ

Muscle Group Focus _____ Weight _____ Date/Time _____

Stretch ○ Warm-Up _____

Strength Training

Exercise	Set	1	2	3	4	5	6	7
	Reps							
	Weight							
	Reps							
	Weight							
	Reps							
	Weight							
	Reps							
	Weight							
	Reps							
	Weight							
	Reps							
	Weight							
	Reps							
	Weight							
	Reps							
	Weight							

Cardio

Exercise	Calories	Distance	Time

Water intake _____

Cooldown _____

Feeling ☆☆☆☆☆

Notes

Goals for Today _____   (M) (T) (W) (T) (F) (S) (S)

Muscle Group Focus _____ Weight _____ Date/Time _____

Stretch ◯ Warm-Up _____

Strength Training

Exercise	Set	1	2	3	4	5	6	7
	Reps							
	Weight							
	Reps							
	Weight							
	Reps							
	Weight							
	Reps							
	Weight							
	Reps							
	Weight							
	Reps							
	Weight							
	Reps							
	Weight							
	Reps							
	Weight							

Cardio

Exercise	Calories	Distance	Time

Water intake _____

Cooldown _____

Feeling ☆☆☆☆☆

Notes

Goals for Today _____ (M) (T) (W) (T) (F) (S) (S)

Muscle Group Focus _____ Weight _____ Date/Time _____

Stretch ○ Warm-Up _____

Strength Training

Exercise	Set	1	2	3	4	5	6	7
	Reps							
	Weight							
	Reps							
	Weight							
	Reps							
	Weight							
	Reps							
	Weight							
	Reps							
	Weight							
	Reps							
	Weight							
	Reps							
	Weight							
	Reps							
	Weight							

Cardio

Exercise	Calories	Distance	Time

Water intake _____

Cooldown _____

Feeling ☆☆☆☆☆

Notes

Goals for Today_____ (M) (T) (W) (T) (F) (S) (S)

Muscle Group Focus _____ Weight _____ Date/Time_____

Stretch ○ Warm-Up_____

Strength Training

Exercise	Set	1	2	3	4	5	6	7
	Reps							
	Weight							
	Reps							
	Weight							
	Reps							
	Weight							
	Reps							
	Weight							
	Reps							
	Weight							
	Reps							
	Weight							
	Reps							
	Weight							
	Reps							
	Weight							

Cardio

Exercise	Calories	Distance	Time

Water intake _____

Cooldown _____

Feeling ☆☆☆☆☆

Notes

Goals for Today _____ Ⓜ Ⓣ Ⓦ Ⓣ Ⓕ Ⓢ Ⓢ

Muscle Group Focus _____ Weight _____ Date/Time _____

Stretch ○ Warm-Up _____

Strength Training

Exercise	Set	1	2	3	4	5	6	7
	Reps							
	Weight							
	Reps							
	Weight							
	Reps							
	Weight							
	Reps							
	Weight							
	Reps							
	Weight							
	Reps							
	Weight							
	Reps							
	Weight							
	Reps							
	Weight							

Cardio

Exercise	Calories	Distance	Time

Water intake _____

Cooldown _____

Feeling ☆☆☆☆☆

Notes

Goals for Today _____ (M) (T) (W) (T) (F) (S) (S)

Muscle Group Focus _____ Weight _____ Date/Time _____

Stretch ○ Warm-Up _____

Strength Training

Exercise	Set	1	2	3	4	5	6	7
	Reps							
	Weight							
	Reps							
	Weight							
	Reps							
	Weight							
	Reps							
	Weight							
	Reps							
	Weight							
	Reps							
	Weight							
	Reps							
	Weight							
	Reps							
	Weight							

Cardio

Exercise	Calories	Distance	Time

Water intake _____

Cooldown _____

Feeling ☆☆☆☆☆

Notes

Goals for Today_____ Ⓜ Ⓣ Ⓦ Ⓣ Ⓕ Ⓢ Ⓢ

Muscle Group Focus _____ Weight _____ Date/Time_____

Stretch ◯ Warm-Up_____

Strength Training

Exercise	Set	1	2	3	4	5	6	7
	Reps							
	Weight							
	Reps							
	Weight							
	Reps							
	Weight							
	Reps							
	Weight							
	Reps							
	Weight							
	Reps							
	Weight							
	Reps							
	Weight							
	Reps							
	Weight							

Cardio

Exercise	Calories	Distance	Time

Water intake _____

Cooldown _____

Feeling ☆☆☆☆☆

Notes

Body Measurement

Date/Period							
Weight							
Body Fat %							
Neck							
Shoulders							
Chest							
Bicep Right							
Bicep Left							
Forearm Right							
Forearm Left							
Wrist							
Waist							
Hips							
Thigh Right							
Thigh Left							
Calf Right							
Calf Left							

Goals

Description	Deadline

Goals for Today _____ (M) (T) (W) (T) (F) (S) (S)

Muscle Group Focus _____ Weight _____ Date/Time _____

Stretch ○ Warm-Up _____

Strength Training

Exercise	Set	1	2	3	4	5	6	7
	Reps							
	Weight							
	Reps							
	Weight							
	Reps							
	Weight							
	Reps							
	Weight							
	Reps							
	Weight							
	Reps							
	Weight							
	Reps							
	Weight							
	Reps							
	Weight							

Cardio

Exercise	Calories	Distance	Time

Water intake _____

Cooldown _____

Feeling ☆☆☆☆☆

Notes

Goals for Today _____ Ⓜ Ⓣ Ⓦ Ⓣ Ⓕ Ⓢ Ⓢ

Muscle Group Focus _____ Weight _____ Date/Time _____

Stretch ○ Warm-Up _____

Strength Training

Exercise	Set	1	2	3	4	5	6	7
	Reps							
	Weight							
	Reps							
	Weight							
	Reps							
	Weight							
	Reps							
	Weight							
	Reps							
	Weight							
	Reps							
	Weight							
	Reps							
	Weight							
	Reps							
	Weight							

Cardio

Exercise	Calories	Distance	Time

Water intake _____

Cooldown _____

Feeling ☆☆☆☆☆

Notes

Goals for Today _____   (M) (T) (W) (T) (F) (S) (S)

Muscle Group Focus _____ Weight _____ Date/Time _____

Stretch ○ Warm-Up _____

Strength Training

Exercise	Set	1	2	3	4	5	6	7
	Reps							
	Weight							
	Reps							
	Weight							
	Reps							
	Weight							
	Reps							
	Weight							
	Reps							
	Weight							
	Reps							
	Weight							
	Reps							
	Weight							
	Reps							
	Weight							

Cardio

Exercise	Calories	Distance	Time
_____			
_____			
_____			
_____			

Water intake _____

Cooldown _____

Feeling ☆☆☆☆☆

Notes

Goals for Today _____   Ⓜ Ⓣ Ⓦ Ⓣ Ⓕ Ⓢ Ⓢ

Muscle Group Focus _____ Weight _____ Date/Time _____

Stretch ○ Warm-Up _____

Strength Training

Exercise	Set	1	2	3	4	5	6	7
	Reps							
	Weight							
	Reps							
	Weight							
	Reps							
	Weight							
	Reps							
	Weight							
	Reps							
	Weight							
	Reps							
	Weight							
	Reps							
	Weight							
	Reps							
	Weight							

Cardio

Exercise	Calories	Distance	Time

Water intake _____

Cooldown _____

Feeling ☆☆☆☆☆

Notes

Goals for Today _____ (M) (T) (W) (T) (F) (S) (S)

Muscle Group Focus _____ Weight _____ Date/Time _____

Stretch ○ Warm-Up _____

Strength Training

Exercise	Set	1	2	3	4	5	6	7
	Reps							
	Weight							
	Reps							
	Weight							
	Reps							
	Weight							
	Reps							
	Weight							
	Reps							
	Weight							
	Reps							
	Weight							
	Reps							
	Weight							
	Reps							
	Weight							

Cardio

Exercise	Calories	Distance	Time

Water intake _____

Cooldown _____

Feeling ☆☆☆☆☆

Notes

Goals for Today _____ Ⓜ Ⓣ Ⓦ Ⓣ Ⓕ Ⓢ Ⓢ

Muscle Group Focus _____ Weight _____ Date/Time _____

Stretch ○ Warm-Up _____

Strength Training

Exercise	Set	1	2	3	4	5	6	7
	Reps							
	Weight							
	Reps							
	Weight							
	Reps							
	Weight							
	Reps							
	Weight							
	Reps							
	Weight							
	Reps							
	Weight							
	Reps							
	Weight							
	Reps							
	Weight							

Cardio

Exercise	Calories	Distance	Time

Water intake _____

Cooldown _____

Feeling ☆☆☆☆☆

Notes

Goals for Today _____ (M) (T) (W) (T) (F) (S) (S)

Muscle Group Focus _____ Weight _____ Date/Time _____

Stretch ○ Warm-Up _____

Strength Training

Exercise	Set	1	2	3	4	5	6	7
	Reps							
	Weight							
	Reps							
	Weight							
	Reps							
	Weight							
	Reps							
	Weight							
	Reps							
	Weight							
	Reps							
	Weight							
	Reps							
	Weight							
	Reps							
	Weight							

Cardio

Exercise	Calories	Distance	Time

Water intake _____

Cooldown _____

Feeling ☆☆☆☆☆

Notes

Goals for Today _____   Ⓜ Ⓣ Ⓦ Ⓣ Ⓕ Ⓢ Ⓢ

Muscle Group Focus _____   Weight _____   Date/Time _____

Stretch ○ Warm-Up _____

Strength Training

Exercise	Set	1	2	3	4	5	6	7
	Reps							
	Weight							
	Reps							
	Weight							
	Reps							
	Weight							
	Reps							
	Weight							
	Reps							
	Weight							
	Reps							
	Weight							
	Reps							
	Weight							
	Reps							
	Weight							

Cardio

Exercise	Calories	Distance	Time

Water intake _____

Cooldown _____

Feeling ☆☆☆☆☆

Notes

Goals for Today _____   Ⓜ Ⓣ Ⓦ Ⓣ Ⓕ Ⓢ Ⓢ

Muscle Group Focus _____ Weight _____ Date/Time _____

Stretch ○ Warm-Up _____

Strength Training

Exercise	Set	1	2	3	4	5	6	7
	Reps							
	Weight							
	Reps							
	Weight							
	Reps							
	Weight							
	Reps							
	Weight							
	Reps							
	Weight							
	Reps							
	Weight							
	Reps							
	Weight							
	Reps							
	Weight							

Cardio

Exercise	Calories	Distance	Time
_____			
_____			
_____			
_____			

Water intake _____

Cooldown _____

Feeling ☆☆☆☆☆

Notes

Goals for Today _____   Ⓜ Ⓣ Ⓦ Ⓣ Ⓕ Ⓢ Ⓢ

Muscle Group Focus _____   Weight _____   Date/Time _____

Stretch ◯   Warm-Up _____

Strength Training

Exercise	Set	1	2	3	4	5	6	7
	Reps							
	Weight							
	Reps							
	Weight							
	Reps							
	Weight							
	Reps							
	Weight							
	Reps							
	Weight							
	Reps							
	Weight							
	Reps							
	Weight							
	Reps							
	Weight							

Cardio

Exercise	Calories	Distance	Time

Water intake _____

Cooldown _____

Feeling ☆☆☆☆☆

Notes

Body Measurement

Date/Period							
Weight							
Body Fat %							
Neck							
Shoulders							
Chest							
Bicep Right							
Bicep Left							
Forearm Right							
Forearm Left							
Wrist							
Waist							
Hips							
Thigh Right							
Thigh Left							
Calf Right							
Calf Left							

Goals

Description	Deadline

Goals for Today _____ (M) (T) (W) (T) (F) (S) (S)

Muscle Group Focus _____ Weight _____ Date/Time _____

Stretch ○ Warm-Up _____

Strength Training

Exercise	Set	1	2	3	4	5	6	7
	Reps							
	Weight							
	Reps							
	Weight							
	Reps							
	Weight							
	Reps							
	Weight							
	Reps							
	Weight							
	Reps							
	Weight							
	Reps							
	Weight							
	Reps							
	Weight							

Cardio

Exercise	Calories	Distance	Time

Water intake _____

Cooldown _____

Feeling ☆☆☆☆☆

Notes

Goals for Today _____   (M) (T) (W) (T) (F) (S) (S)

Muscle Group Focus _____   Weight _____   Date/Time _____

Stretch ◯ Warm-Up _____

Strength Training

Exercise	Set	1	2	3	4	5	6	7
	Reps							
	Weight							
	Reps							
	Weight							
	Reps							
	Weight							
	Reps							
	Weight							
	Reps							
	Weight							
	Reps							
	Weight							
	Reps							
	Weight							
	Reps							
	Weight							

Cardio

Exercise	Calories	Distance	Time
_____			
_____			
_____			
_____			

Water intake _____

Cooldown _____

Feeling ☆☆☆☆☆

Notes

Goals for Today _____ (M) (T) (W) (T) (F) (S) (S)

Muscle Group Focus _____ Weight _____ Date/Time _____

Stretch ◯ Warm-Up _____

Strength Training

Exercise	Set	1	2	3	4	5	6	7
	Reps							
	Weight							
	Reps							
	Weight							
	Reps							
	Weight							
	Reps							
	Weight							
	Reps							
	Weight							
	Reps							
	Weight							
	Reps							
	Weight							
	Reps							
	Weight							

Cardio

Exercise	Calories	Distance	Time
_____			
_____			
_____			
_____			

Water intake _____

Cooldown _____

Feeling ☆☆☆☆☆

Notes

Goals for Today _____   (M) (T) (W) (T) (F) (S) (S)

Muscle Group Focus _____ Weight _____ Date/Time _____

Stretch ○ Warm-Up _____

Strength Training

Exercise	Set	1	2	3	4	5	6	7
	Reps							
	Weight							
	Reps							
	Weight							
	Reps							
	Weight							
	Reps							
	Weight							
	Reps							
	Weight							
	Reps							
	Weight							
	Reps							
	Weight							
	Reps							
	Weight							

Cardio

Exercise	Calories	Distance	Time

Water intake _____

Cooldown _____

Feeling ☆☆☆☆☆

Notes

Goals for Today _____   (M) (T) (W) (T) (F) (S) (S)

Muscle Group Focus _____ Weight _____ Date/Time _____

Stretch ○ Warm-Up _____

Strength Training

Exercise	Set	1	2	3	4	5	6	7
	Reps							
	Weight							
	Reps							
	Weight							
	Reps							
	Weight							
	Reps							
	Weight							
	Reps							
	Weight							
	Reps							
	Weight							
	Reps							
	Weight							
	Reps							
	Weight							

Cardio

Exercise	Calories	Distance	Time
_____			
_____			
_____			
_____			

Water intake _____

Cooldown _____

Feeling ☆☆☆☆☆

Notes

Goals for Today _____ Ⓜ Ⓣ Ⓦ Ⓣ Ⓕ Ⓢ Ⓢ

Muscle Group Focus _____ Weight _____ Date/Time _____

Stretch ○ Warm-Up _____

Strength Training

Exercise	Set	1	2	3	4	5	6	7
	Reps							
	Weight							
	Reps							
	Weight							
	Reps							
	Weight							
	Reps							
	Weight							
	Reps							
	Weight							
	Reps							
	Weight							
	Reps							
	Weight							
	Reps							
	Weight							

Cardio

Exercise	Calories	Distance	Time

Water intake _____

Cooldown _____

Feeling ☆☆☆☆☆

Notes

Goals for Today _____   Ⓜ Ⓣ Ⓦ Ⓣ Ⓕ Ⓢ Ⓢ

Muscle Group Focus _____ Weight _____ Date/Time _____

Stretch ◯ Warm-Up _____

Strength Training

Exercise	Set	1	2	3	4	5	6	7
	Reps							
	Weight							
	Reps							
	Weight							
	Reps							
	Weight							
	Reps							
	Weight							
	Reps							
	Weight							
	Reps							
	Weight							
	Reps							
	Weight							
	Reps							
	Weight							

Cardio

Exercise	Calories	Distance	Time

Water intake _____

Cooldown _____

Feeling ☆☆☆☆☆

Notes

Goals for Today_____ Ⓜ Ⓣ Ⓦ Ⓣ Ⓕ Ⓢ Ⓢ

Muscle Group Focus _____ Weight _____ Date/Time_____

Stretch ○ Warm-Up_____

Strength Training

Exercise	Set	1	2	3	4	5	6	7
	Reps							
	Weight							
	Reps							
	Weight							
	Reps							
	Weight							
	Reps							
	Weight							
	Reps							
	Weight							
	Reps							
	Weight							
	Reps							
	Weight							
	Reps							
	Weight							

Cardio

Exercise	Calories	Distance	Time

Water intake _____

Cooldown _____

Feeling ☆☆☆☆☆

Notes

Goals for Today _____   (M) (T) (W) (T) (F) (S) (S)

Muscle Group Focus _____ Weight _____ Date/Time _____

Stretch ○ Warm-Up _____

Strength Training

Exercise	Set	1	2	3	4	5	6	7
	Reps							
	Weight							
	Reps							
	Weight							
	Reps							
	Weight							
	Reps							
	Weight							
	Reps							
	Weight							
	Reps							
	Weight							
	Reps							
	Weight							
	Reps							
	Weight							

Cardio

Exercise	Calories	Distance	Time

Water intake _____

Cooldown _____

Feeling ☆☆☆☆☆

Notes

Goals for Today _____   (M) (T) (W) (T) (F) (S) (S)

Muscle Group Focus _____   Weight _____   Date/Time _____

Stretch ◯   Warm-Up _____

Strength Training

Exercise	Set	1	2	3	4	5	6	7
	Reps							
	Weight							
	Reps							
	Weight							
	Reps							
	Weight							
	Reps							
	Weight							
	Reps							
	Weight							
	Reps							
	Weight							
	Reps							
	Weight							
	Reps							
	Weight							

Cardio

Exercise	Calories	Distance	Time

Water intake _____

Cooldown _____

Feeling ☆☆☆☆☆

Notes

Body Measurement

Date/Period							
Weight							
Body Fat %							
Neck							
Shoulders							
Chest							
Bicep Right							
Bicep Left							
Forearm Right							
Forearm Left							
Wrist							
Waist							
Hips							
Thigh Right							
Thigh Left							
Calf Right							
Calf Left							

Goals

Description	Deadline

Goals for Today _____ Ⓜ Ⓣ Ⓦ Ⓣ Ⓕ Ⓢ Ⓢ

Muscle Group Focus _____ Weight _____ Date/Time _____

Stretch ◯ Warm-Up _____

Strength Training

Exercise	Set	1	2	3	4	5	6	7
	Reps							
	Weight							
	Reps							
	Weight							
	Reps							
	Weight							
	Reps							
	Weight							
	Reps							
	Weight							
	Reps							
	Weight							
	Reps							
	Weight							
	Reps							
	Weight							

Cardio

Exercise	Calories	Distance	Time
_____			
_____			
_____			

Water intake _____

Cooldown _____

Feeling ☆☆☆☆☆

Notes

Goals for Today _____ Ⓜ Ⓣ Ⓦ Ⓣ Ⓕ Ⓢ Ⓢ

Muscle Group Focus _____ Weight _____ Date/Time _____

Stretch ○ Warm-Up _____

Strength Training

Exercise	Set	1	2	3	4	5	6	7
	Reps							
	Weight							
	Reps							
	Weight							
	Reps							
	Weight							
	Reps							
	Weight							
	Reps							
	Weight							
	Reps							
	Weight							
	Reps							
	Weight							
	Reps							
	Weight							

Cardio

Exercise	Calories	Distance	Time

Water intake _____

Cooldown _____

Feeling ☆☆☆☆☆

Notes

Goals for Today _____ (M) (T) (W) (T) (F) (S) (S)

Muscle Group Focus _____ Weight _____ Date/Time _____

Stretch ○ Warm-Up _____

Strength Training

Exercise	Set	1	2	3	4	5	6	7
	Reps							
	Weight							
	Reps							
	Weight							
	Reps							
	Weight							
	Reps							
	Weight							
	Reps							
	Weight							
	Reps							
	Weight							
	Reps							
	Weight							
	Reps							
	Weight							

Cardio

Exercise	Calories	Distance	Time

Water intake _____

Cooldown _____

Feeling ☆☆☆☆☆

Notes

Goals for Today _____   (M) (T) (W) (T) (F) (S) (S)

Muscle Group Focus _____   Weight _____   Date/Time _____

Stretch ◯   Warm-Up _____

Strength Training

Exercise	Set	1	2	3	4	5	6	7
	Reps							
	Weight							
	Reps							
	Weight							
	Reps							
	Weight							
	Reps							
	Weight							
	Reps							
	Weight							
	Reps							
	Weight							
	Reps							
	Weight							
	Reps							
	Weight							

Cardio

Exercise	Calories	Distance	Time

Water intake _____

Cooldown _____

Feeling ☆☆☆☆☆

Notes

Goals for Today _____ Ⓜ Ⓣ Ⓦ Ⓣ Ⓕ Ⓢ Ⓢ

Muscle Group Focus _____ Weight _____ Date/Time _____

Stretch ◯ Warm-Up _____

Strength Training

Exercise	Set	1	2	3	4	5	6	7
	Reps							
	Weight							
	Reps							
	Weight							
	Reps							
	Weight							
	Reps							
	Weight							
	Reps							
	Weight							
	Reps							
	Weight							
	Reps							
	Weight							
	Reps							
	Weight							

Cardio

Exercise	Calories	Distance	Time

Water intake _____

Cooldown _____

Feeling ☆☆☆☆☆

Notes

Goals for Today _____ Ⓜ Ⓣ Ⓦ Ⓣ Ⓕ Ⓢ Ⓢ

Muscle Group Focus _____ Weight _____ Date/Time _____

Stretch ○ Warm-Up _____

Strength Training

Exercise	Set	1	2	3	4	5	6	7
	Reps							
	Weight							
	Reps							
	Weight							
	Reps							
	Weight							
	Reps							
	Weight							
	Reps							
	Weight							
	Reps							
	Weight							
	Reps							
	Weight							
	Reps							
	Weight							

Cardio

Exercise	Calories	Distance	Time
_____			
_____			
_____			
_____			

Water intake _____

Cooldown _____

Feeling ☆☆☆☆☆

Notes

Goals for Today _____   (M) (T) (W) (T) (F) (S) (S)

Muscle Group Focus _____ Weight _____ Date/Time _____

Stretch ◯ Warm-Up_____

Strength Training

Exercise	Set	1	2	3	4	5	6	7
	Reps							
	Weight							
	Reps							
	Weight							
	Reps							
	Weight							
	Reps							
	Weight							
	Reps							
	Weight							
	Reps							
	Weight							
	Reps							
	Weight							
	Reps							
	Weight							

Cardio

Exercise	Calories	Distance	Time

Water intake _____

Cooldown _____

Feeling ☆☆☆☆☆

Notes

Goals for Today _____   Ⓜ Ⓣ Ⓦ Ⓣ Ⓕ Ⓢ Ⓢ

Muscle Group Focus _____   Weight _____   Date/Time _____

Stretch ◯   Warm-Up _____

Strength Training

Exercise	Set	1	2	3	4	5	6	7
	Reps							
	Weight							
	Reps							
	Weight							
	Reps							
	Weight							
	Reps							
	Weight							
	Reps							
	Weight							
	Reps							
	Weight							
	Reps							
	Weight							
	Reps							
	Weight							

Cardio

Exercise	Calories	Distance	Time

Water intake _____

Cooldown _____

Feeling ☆☆☆☆☆

Notes

Goals for Today _____ (M) (T) (W) (T) (F) (S) (S)

Muscle Group Focus _____ Weight _____ Date/Time _____

Stretch ◯ Warm-Up _____

Strength Training

Exercise	Set	1	2	3	4	5	6	7
	Reps							
	Weight							
	Reps							
	Weight							
	Reps							
	Weight							
	Reps							
	Weight							
	Reps							
	Weight							
	Reps							
	Weight							
	Reps							
	Weight							
	Reps							
	Weight							

Cardio

Exercise	Calories	Distance	Time
_____			
_____			
_____			
_____			

Water intake _____

Cooldown _____

Feeling ☆☆☆☆☆

Notes

Goals for Today _____ Ⓜ Ⓣ Ⓦ Ⓣ Ⓕ Ⓢ Ⓢ

Muscle Group Focus _____ Weight _____ Date/Time _____

Stretch ○ Warm-Up _____

Strength Training

Exercise	Set	1	2	3	4	5	6	7
	Reps							
	Weight							
	Reps							
	Weight							
	Reps							
	Weight							
	Reps							
	Weight							
	Reps							
	Weight							
	Reps							
	Weight							
	Reps							
	Weight							
	Reps							
	Weight							

Cardio

Exercise	Calories	Distance	Time

Water intake _____

Cooldown _____

Feeling ☆☆☆☆☆

Notes

Body Measurement

Date/Period							
Weight							
Body Fat %							
Neck							
Shoulders							
Chest							
Bicep Right							
Bicep Left							
Forearm Right							
Forearm Left							
Wrist							
Waist							
Hips							
Thigh Right							
Thigh Left							
Calf Right							
Calf Left							

Goals

Description	Deadline

Goals for Today _____ (M) (T) (W) (T) (F) (S) (S)

Muscle Group Focus _____ Weight _____ Date/Time _____

Stretch ◯ Warm-Up _____

Strength Training

Exercise	Set	1	2	3	4	5	6	7
	Reps							
	Weight							
	Reps							
	Weight							
	Reps							
	Weight							
	Reps							
	Weight							
	Reps							
	Weight							
	Reps							
	Weight							
	Reps							
	Weight							
	Reps							
	Weight							

Cardio

Exercise	Calories	Distance	Time
_____			
_____			
_____			

Water intake _____

Cooldown _____

Feeling ☆☆☆☆☆

Notes

Goals for Today_____ Ⓜ Ⓣ Ⓦ Ⓣ Ⓕ Ⓢ Ⓢ

Muscle Group Focus _____ Weight _____ Date/Time_____

Stretch ○ Warm-Up_____

Strength Training

Exercise	Set	1	2	3	4	5	6	7
	Reps							
	Weight							
	Reps							
	Weight							
	Reps							
	Weight							
	Reps							
	Weight							
	Reps							
	Weight							
	Reps							
	Weight							
	Reps							
	Weight							
	Reps							
	Weight							

Cardio

Exercise	Calories	Distance	Time

Water intake _____

Cooldown _____

Feeling ☆☆☆☆☆

Notes

Goals for Today_____   (M) (T) (W) (T) (F) (S) (S)

Muscle Group Focus _____ Weight _____ Date/Time_____

Stretch ◯ Warm-Up_____

Strength Training

Exercise	Set	1	2	3	4	5	6	7
	Reps							
	Weight							
	Reps							
	Weight							
	Reps							
	Weight							
	Reps							
	Weight							
	Reps							
	Weight							
	Reps							
	Weight							
	Reps							
	Weight							
	Reps							
	Weight							

Cardio

Exercise	Calories	Distance	Time
_____			
_____			
_____			
_____			

Water intake _____

Cooldown _____

Feeling ☆☆☆☆☆

Notes

Goals for Today _____ Ⓜ Ⓣ Ⓦ Ⓣ Ⓕ Ⓢ Ⓢ

Muscle Group Focus _____ Weight _____ Date/Time _____

Stretch ◯ Warm-Up _____

Strength Training

Exercise	Set	1	2	3	4	5	6	7
	Reps							
	Weight							
	Reps							
	Weight							
	Reps							
	Weight							
	Reps							
	Weight							
	Reps							
	Weight							
	Reps							
	Weight							
	Reps							
	Weight							
	Reps							
	Weight							

Cardio

Exercise	Calories	Distance	Time

Water intake _____

Cooldown _____

Feeling ☆☆☆☆☆

Notes

Goals for Today _____ Ⓜ Ⓣ Ⓦ Ⓣ Ⓕ Ⓢ Ⓢ

Muscle Group Focus _____ Weight _____ Date/Time _____

Stretch ○ Warm-Up _____

Strength Training

Exercise	Set	1	2	3	4	5	6	7
	Reps							
	Weight							
	Reps							
	Weight							
	Reps							
	Weight							
	Reps							
	Weight							
	Reps							
	Weight							
	Reps							
	Weight							
	Reps							
	Weight							
	Reps							
	Weight							

Cardio

Exercise	Calories	Distance	Time
_____			
_____			
_____			
_____			

Water intake _____

Cooldown _____

Feeling ☆☆☆☆☆

Notes

Goals for Today _____   Ⓜ Ⓣ Ⓦ Ⓣ Ⓕ Ⓢ Ⓢ

Muscle Group Focus _____ Weight _____ Date/Time _____

Stretch ○ Warm-Up _____

Strength Training

Exercise	Set	1	2	3	4	5	6	7
	Reps							
	Weight							
	Reps							
	Weight							
	Reps							
	Weight							
	Reps							
	Weight							
	Reps							
	Weight							
	Reps							
	Weight							
	Reps							
	Weight							
	Reps							
	Weight							

Cardio

Exercise	Calories	Distance	Time

Water intake _____

Cooldown _____

Feeling ☆☆☆☆☆

Notes

Goals for Today _____   Ⓜ Ⓣ Ⓦ Ⓣ Ⓕ Ⓢ Ⓢ

Muscle Group Focus _____ Weight _____ Date/Time _____

Stretch ◯ Warm-Up _____

Strength Training

Exercise	Set	1	2	3	4	5	6	7
	Reps							
	Weight							
	Reps							
	Weight							
	Reps							
	Weight							
	Reps							
	Weight							
	Reps							
	Weight							
	Reps							
	Weight							
	Reps							
	Weight							
	Reps							
	Weight							

Cardio

Exercise	Calories	Distance	Time

Water intake _____

Cooldown _____

Feeling ☆☆☆☆☆

Notes

Goals for Today _____ (M) (T) (W) (T) (F) (S) (S)

Muscle Group Focus _____ Weight _____ Date/Time _____

Stretch ○ Warm-Up _____

Strength Training

Exercise	Set	1	2	3	4	5	6	7
	Reps							
	Weight							
	Reps							
	Weight							
	Reps							
	Weight							
	Reps							
	Weight							
	Reps							
	Weight							
	Reps							
	Weight							
	Reps							
	Weight							
	Reps							
	Weight							

Cardio

Exercise	Calories	Distance	Time

Water intake _____

Cooldown _____

Feeling ☆☆☆☆☆

Notes

Goals for Today _____   (M) (T) (W) (T) (F) (S) (S)

Muscle Group Focus _____ Weight _____ Date/Time _____

Stretch ⚪ Warm-Up _____

Strength Training

Exercise	Set	1	2	3	4	5	6	7
	Reps							
	Weight							
	Reps							
	Weight							
	Reps							
	Weight							
	Reps							
	Weight							
	Reps							
	Weight							
	Reps							
	Weight							
	Reps							
	Weight							
	Reps							
	Weight							

Cardio

Exercise	Calories	Distance	Time
_____			
_____			
_____			

Water intake _____

Cooldown _____

Feeling ☆☆☆☆☆

Notes

Goals for Today _____ (M) (T) (W) (T) (F) (S) (S)

Muscle Group Focus _____ Weight _____ Date/Time _____

Stretch ○ Warm-Up _____

Strength Training

Exercise	Set	1	2	3	4	5	6	7
	Reps							
	Weight							
	Reps							
	Weight							
	Reps							
	Weight							
	Reps							
	Weight							
	Reps							
	Weight							
	Reps							
	Weight							
	Reps							
	Weight							
	Reps							
	Weight							

Cardio

Exercise	Calories	Distance	Time

Water intake _____

Cooldown _____

Feeling ☆☆☆☆☆

Notes

Body Measurement

Date/Period							
Weight							
Body Fat %							
Neck							
Shoulders							
Chest							
Bicep Right							
Bicep Left							
Forearm Right							
Forearm Left							
Wrist							
Waist							
Hips							
Thigh Right							
Thigh Left							
Calf Right							
Calf Left							

Goals

Description	Deadline

Goals for Today _____ Ⓜ Ⓣ Ⓦ Ⓣ Ⓕ Ⓢ Ⓢ

Muscle Group Focus _____ Weight _____ Date/Time _____

Stretch ◯ Warm-Up _____

Strength Training

Exercise	Set	1	2	3	4	5	6	7
	Reps							
	Weight							
	Reps							
	Weight							
	Reps							
	Weight							
	Reps							
	Weight							
	Reps							
	Weight							
	Reps							
	Weight							
	Reps							
	Weight							
	Reps							
	Weight							

Cardio

Exercise	Calories	Distance	Time

Water intake _____

Cooldown _____

Feeling ☆☆☆☆☆

Notes

Goals for Today _____   Ⓜ Ⓣ Ⓦ Ⓣ Ⓕ Ⓢ Ⓢ

Muscle Group Focus _____   Weight _____   Date/Time _____

Stretch ○   Warm-Up _____

Strength Training

Exercise	Set	1	2	3	4	5	6	7
	Reps							
	Weight							
	Reps							
	Weight							
	Reps							
	Weight							
	Reps							
	Weight							
	Reps							
	Weight							
	Reps							
	Weight							
	Reps							
	Weight							
	Reps							
	Weight							

Cardio

Exercise	Calories	Distance	Time
_____			
_____			
_____			
_____			

Water intake _____

Cooldown _____

Feeling ☆☆☆☆☆

Notes

Goals for Today _____ (M) (T) (W) (T) (F) (S) (S)

Muscle Group Focus _____ Weight _____ Date/Time _____

Stretch ◯ Warm-Up _____

Strength Training

Exercise	Set	1	2	3	4	5	6	7
	Reps							
	Weight							
	Reps							
	Weight							
	Reps							
	Weight							
	Reps							
	Weight							
	Reps							
	Weight							
	Reps							
	Weight							
	Reps							
	Weight							
	Reps							
	Weight							

Cardio

Exercise	Calories	Distance	Time

Water intake _____

Cooldown _____

Feeling ☆☆☆☆☆

Notes

Goals for Today _____ Ⓜ Ⓣ Ⓦ Ⓣ Ⓕ Ⓢ Ⓢ

Muscle Group Focus _____ Weight _____ Date/Time _____

Stretch ◯ Warm-Up _____

Strength Training

Exercise	Set	1	2	3	4	5	6	7
	Reps							
	Weight							
	Reps							
	Weight							
	Reps							
	Weight							
	Reps							
	Weight							
	Reps							
	Weight							
	Reps							
	Weight							
	Reps							
	Weight							
	Reps							
	Weight							

Cardio

Exercise	Calories	Distance	Time
_____			
_____			
_____			
_____			

Water intake _____

Cooldown _____

Feeling ☆☆☆☆☆

Notes

Goals for Today _____ Ⓜ Ⓣ Ⓦ Ⓣ Ⓕ Ⓢ Ⓢ

Muscle Group Focus _____ Weight _____ Date/Time _____

Stretch ○ Warm-Up _____

Strength Training

Exercise	Set	1	2	3	4	5	6	7
	Reps							
	Weight							
	Reps							
	Weight							
	Reps							
	Weight							
	Reps							
	Weight							
	Reps							
	Weight							
	Reps							
	Weight							
	Reps							
	Weight							
	Reps							
	Weight							

Cardio

Exercise	Calories	Distance	Time
_____			
_____			
_____			
_____			

Water intake _____

Cooldown _____

Feeling ☆☆☆☆☆

Notes

Goals for Today _____ Ⓜ Ⓣ Ⓦ Ⓣ Ⓕ Ⓢ Ⓢ

Muscle Group Focus _____ Weight _____ Date/Time _____

Stretch ○ Warm-Up _____

Strength Training

Exercise	Set	1	2	3	4	5	6	7
	Reps							
	Weight							
	Reps							
	Weight							
	Reps							
	Weight							
	Reps							
	Weight							
	Reps							
	Weight							
	Reps							
	Weight							
	Reps							
	Weight							
	Reps							
	Weight							

Cardio

Exercise	Calories	Distance	Time
_____			
_____			
_____			
_____			

Water intake _____

Cooldown _____

Feeling ☆☆☆☆☆

Notes

Goals for Today _____   Ⓜ Ⓣ Ⓦ Ⓣ Ⓕ Ⓢ Ⓢ

Muscle Group Focus _____ Weight _____ Date/Time _____

Stretch ◯ Warm-Up _____

Strength Training

Exercise	Set	1	2	3	4	5	6	7
	Reps							
	Weight							
	Reps							
	Weight							
	Reps							
	Weight							
	Reps							
	Weight							
	Reps							
	Weight							
	Reps							
	Weight							
	Reps							
	Weight							
	Reps							
	Weight							

Cardio

Exercise	Calories	Distance	Time
_____			
_____			
_____			
_____			

Water intake _____

Cooldown _____

Feeling ☆☆☆☆☆

Notes

Goals for Today _____ (M) (T) (W) (T) (F) (S) (S)

Muscle Group Focus _____ Weight _____ Date/Time _____

Stretch ◯ Warm-Up _____

Strength Training

Exercise	Set	1	2	3	4	5	6	7
	Reps							
	Weight							
	Reps							
	Weight							
	Reps							
	Weight							
	Reps							
	Weight							
	Reps							
	Weight							
	Reps							
	Weight							
	Reps							
	Weight							
	Reps							
	Weight							

Cardio

Exercise	Calories	Distance	Time
_____			
_____			
_____			
_____			

Water intake _____

Cooldown _____

Feeling ☆☆☆☆☆

Notes

Goals for Today _____   (M) (T) (W) (T) (F) (S) (S)

Muscle Group Focus _____ Weight _____ Date/Time _____

Stretch ○ Warm-Up _____

Strength Training

Exercise	Set	1	2	3	4	5	6	7
	Reps							
	Weight							
	Reps							
	Weight							
	Reps							
	Weight							
	Reps							
	Weight							
	Reps							
	Weight							
	Reps							
	Weight							
	Reps							
	Weight							
	Reps							
	Weight							

Cardio

Exercise	Calories	Distance	Time
_____			
_____			
_____			
_____			

Water intake _____

Cooldown _____

Feeling ☆☆☆☆☆

Notes

Goals for Today _____   Ⓜ Ⓣ Ⓦ Ⓣ Ⓕ Ⓢ Ⓢ

Muscle Group Focus _____ Weight _____ Date/Time _____

Stretch ○ Warm-Up _____

Strength Training

Exercise	Set	1	2	3	4	5	6	7
	Reps							
	Weight							
	Reps							
	Weight							
	Reps							
	Weight							
	Reps							
	Weight							
	Reps							
	Weight							
	Reps							
	Weight							
	Reps							
	Weight							
	Reps							
	Weight							

Cardio

Exercise	Calories	Distance	Time

Water intake _____

Cooldown _____

Feeling ☆☆☆☆☆

Notes

Body Measurement

Date/Period							
Weight							
Body Fat %							
Neck							
Shoulders							
Chest							
Bicep Right							
Bicep Left							
Forearm Right							
Forearm Left							
Wrist							
Waist							
Hips							
Thigh Right							
Thigh Left							
Calf Right							
Calf Left							

Goals

Description	Deadline

Goals for Today _____ (M) (T) (W) (T) (F) (S) (S)

Muscle Group Focus _____ Weight _____ Date/Time _____

Stretch ○ Warm-Up _____

Strength Training

Exercise	Set	1	2	3	4	5	6	7
	Reps							
	Weight							
	Reps							
	Weight							
	Reps							
	Weight							
	Reps							
	Weight							
	Reps							
	Weight							
	Reps							
	Weight							
	Reps							
	Weight							
	Reps							
	Weight							

Cardio

Exercise	Calories	Distance	Time

Water intake _____

Cooldown _____

Feeling ☆☆☆☆☆

Notes

Goals for Today _____ (M) (T) (W) (T) (F) (S) (S)

Muscle Group Focus _____ Weight _____ Date/Time _____

Stretch ○ Warm-Up _____

Strength Training

Exercise	Set	1	2	3	4	5	6	7
	Reps							
	Weight							
	Reps							
	Weight							
	Reps							
	Weight							
	Reps							
	Weight							
	Reps							
	Weight							
	Reps							
	Weight							
	Reps							
	Weight							
	Reps							
	Weight							

Cardio

Exercise	Calories	Distance	Time

Water intake _____

Cooldown _____

Feeling ☆☆☆☆☆

Notes

Goals for Today _____   Ⓜ Ⓣ Ⓦ Ⓣ Ⓕ Ⓢ Ⓢ

Muscle Group Focus _____ Weight _____ Date/Time _____

Stretch ◯ Warm-Up _____

Strength Training

Exercise	Set	1	2	3	4	5	6	7
	Reps							
	Weight							
	Reps							
	Weight							
	Reps							
	Weight							
	Reps							
	Weight							
	Reps							
	Weight							
	Reps							
	Weight							
	Reps							
	Weight							
	Reps							
	Weight							

Cardio

Exercise	Calories	Distance	Time
_____			
_____			
_____			
_____			

Water intake _____

Cooldown _____

Feeling ☆☆☆☆☆

Notes

Goals for Today _____   Ⓜ Ⓣ Ⓦ Ⓣ Ⓕ Ⓢ Ⓢ

Muscle Group Focus _____   Weight _____   Date/Time _____

Stretch ◯   Warm-Up _____

Strength Training

Exercise	Set	1	2	3	4	5	6	7
	Reps							
	Weight							
	Reps							
	Weight							
	Reps							
	Weight							
	Reps							
	Weight							
	Reps							
	Weight							
	Reps							
	Weight							
	Reps							
	Weight							
	Reps							
	Weight							

Cardio

Exercise	Calories	Distance	Time
_____			
_____			
_____			
_____			

Water intake _____

Cooldown _____

Feeling ☆☆☆☆☆

Notes

Goals for Today _____ (M) (T) (W) (T) (F) (S) (S)

Muscle Group Focus _____ Weight _____ Date/Time _____

Stretch ○ Warm-Up _____

Strength Training

Exercise	Set	1	2	3	4	5	6	7
	Reps							
	Weight							
	Reps							
	Weight							
	Reps							
	Weight							
	Reps							
	Weight							
	Reps							
	Weight							
	Reps							
	Weight							
	Reps							
	Weight							
	Reps							
	Weight							

Cardio

Exercise	Calories	Distance	Time
_____			
_____			
_____			
_____			

Water intake _____

Cooldown _____

Feeling ☆☆☆☆☆

Notes

Goals for Today _____ (M) (T) (W) (T) (F) (S) (S)

Muscle Group Focus _____ Weight _____ Date/Time _____

Stretch ○ Warm-Up _____

Strength Training

Exercise	Set	1	2	3	4	5	6	7
	Reps							
	Weight							
	Reps							
	Weight							
	Reps							
	Weight							
	Reps							
	Weight							
	Reps							
	Weight							
	Reps							
	Weight							
	Reps							
	Weight							
	Reps							
	Weight							

Cardio

Exercise	Calories	Distance	Time
_____			
_____			
_____			
_____			

Water intake _____

Cooldown _____

Feeling ☆☆☆☆☆

Notes

Goals for Today _____   (M) (T) (W) (T) (F) (S) (S)

Muscle Group Focus _____ Weight _____ Date/Time _____

Stretch ◯ Warm-Up _____

Strength Training

Exercise	Set	1	2	3	4	5	6	7
	Reps							
	Weight							
	Reps							
	Weight							
	Reps							
	Weight							
	Reps							
	Weight							
	Reps							
	Weight							
	Reps							
	Weight							
	Reps							
	Weight							
	Reps							
	Weight							

Cardio

Exercise	Calories	Distance	Time
_____			
_____			
_____			
_____			

Water intake _____

Cooldown _____

Feeling ☆☆☆☆☆

Notes

Goals for Today _____ (M) (T) (W) (T) (F) (S) (S)

Muscle Group Focus _____ Weight _____ Date/Time _____

Stretch ○ Warm-Up _____

Strength Training

Exercise	Set	1	2	3	4	5	6	7
	Reps							
	Weight							
	Reps							
	Weight							
	Reps							
	Weight							
	Reps							
	Weight							
	Reps							
	Weight							
	Reps							
	Weight							
	Reps							
	Weight							
	Reps							
	Weight							

Cardio

Exercise	Calories	Distance	Time

Water intake _____

Cooldown _____

Feeling ☆☆☆☆☆

Notes

Goals for Today _____ (M) (T) (W) (T) (F) (S) (S)

Muscle Group Focus _____ Weight _____ Date/Time _____

Stretch ◯ Warm-Up _____

Strength Training

Exercise	Set	1	2	3	4	5	6	7
	Reps							
	Weight							
	Reps							
	Weight							
	Reps							
	Weight							
	Reps							
	Weight							
	Reps							
	Weight							
	Reps							
	Weight							
	Reps							
	Weight							
	Reps							
	Weight							

Cardio

Exercise	Calories	Distance	Time

Water intake _____

Cooldown _____

Feeling ☆☆☆☆☆

Notes

Goals for Today_____   Ⓜ Ⓣ Ⓦ Ⓣ Ⓕ Ⓢ Ⓢ

Muscle Group Focus_____ Weight_____ Date/Time_____

Stretch ◯ Warm-Up_____

Strength Training

Exercise	Set	1	2	3	4	5	6	7
	Reps							
	Weight							
	Reps							
	Weight							
	Reps							
	Weight							
	Reps							
	Weight							
	Reps							
	Weight							
	Reps							
	Weight							
	Reps							
	Weight							
	Reps							
	Weight							

Cardio

Exercise	Calories	Distance	Time

Water intake _____

Cooldown _____

Feeling ☆☆☆☆☆

Notes

Body Measurement

Date/Period							
Weight							
Body Fat %							
Neck							
Shoulders							
Chest							
Bicep Right							
Bicep Left							
Forearm Right							
Forearm Left							
Wrist							
Waist							
Hips							
Thigh Right							
Thigh Left							
Calf Right							
Calf Left							

Goals

Description	Deadline

Goals for Today _____   (M) (T) (W) (T) (F) (S) (S)

Muscle Group Focus _____ Weight _____ Date/Time _____

Stretch ◯ Warm-Up_____

Strength Training

Exercise	Set	1	2	3	4	5	6	7
	Reps							
	Weight							
	Reps							
	Weight							
	Reps							
	Weight							
	Reps							
	Weight							
	Reps							
	Weight							
	Reps							
	Weight							
	Reps							
	Weight							
	Reps							
	Weight							

Cardio

Exercise	Calories	Distance	Time
_____			
_____			
_____			
_____			

Water intake _____

Cooldown _____

Feeling ☆☆☆☆☆

Notes

Goals for Today _____ Ⓜ Ⓣ Ⓦ Ⓣ Ⓕ Ⓢ Ⓢ

Muscle Group Focus _____ Weight _____ Date/Time _____

Stretch ◯ Warm-Up _____

Strength Training

Exercise	Set	1	2	3	4	5	6	7
	Reps							
	Weight							
	Reps							
	Weight							
	Reps							
	Weight							
	Reps							
	Weight							
	Reps							
	Weight							
	Reps							
	Weight							
	Reps							
	Weight							
	Reps							
	Weight							

Cardio

Exercise	Calories	Distance	Time
_____			
_____			
_____			
_____			

Water intake _____

Cooldown _____

Feeling ☆☆☆☆☆

Notes

Goals for Today _____   Ⓜ Ⓣ Ⓦ Ⓣ Ⓕ Ⓢ Ⓢ

Muscle Group Focus _____   Weight _____   Date/Time _____

Stretch ○   Warm-Up _____

Strength Training

Exercise	Set	1	2	3	4	5	6	7
	Reps							
	Weight							
	Reps							
	Weight							
	Reps							
	Weight							
	Reps							
	Weight							
	Reps							
	Weight							
	Reps							
	Weight							
	Reps							
	Weight							
	Reps							
	Weight							

Cardio

Exercise	Calories	Distance	Time

Water intake _____

Cooldown _____

Feeling ☆☆☆☆☆

Notes

Goals for Today _____ (M) (T) (W) (T) (F) (S) (S)

Muscle Group Focus _____ Weight _____ Date/Time _____

Stretch ○ Warm-Up _____

Strength Training

Exercise	Set	1	2	3	4	5	6	7
	Reps							
	Weight							
	Reps							
	Weight							
	Reps							
	Weight							
	Reps							
	Weight							
	Reps							
	Weight							
	Reps							
	Weight							
	Reps							
	Weight							
	Reps							
	Weight							

Cardio

Exercise	Calories	Distance	Time

Water intake _____

Cooldown _____

Feeling ☆☆☆☆☆

Notes

Goals for Today _____   (M) (T) (W) (T) (F) (S) (S)

Muscle Group Focus _____ Weight _____ Date/Time _____

Stretch ◯ Warm-Up _____

Strength Training

Exercise	Set	1	2	3	4	5	6	7
	Reps							
	Weight							
	Reps							
	Weight							
	Reps							
	Weight							
	Reps							
	Weight							
	Reps							
	Weight							
	Reps							
	Weight							
	Reps							
	Weight							
	Reps							
	Weight							

Cardio

Exercise	Calories	Distance	Time
_____			
_____			
_____			
_____			

Water intake _____

Cooldown _____

Feeling ☆☆☆☆☆

Notes

Goals for Today _____   Ⓜ Ⓣ Ⓦ Ⓣ Ⓕ Ⓢ Ⓢ

Muscle Group Focus _____ Weight _____ Date/Time _____

Stretch ◯ Warm-Up _____

Strength Training

Exercise	Set	1	2	3	4	5	6	7
	Reps							
	Weight							
	Reps							
	Weight							
	Reps							
	Weight							
	Reps							
	Weight							
	Reps							
	Weight							
	Reps							
	Weight							
	Reps							
	Weight							
	Reps							
	Weight							

Cardio

Exercise	Calories	Distance	Time

Water intake _____

Cooldown _____

Feeling ☆☆☆☆☆

Notes

Goals for Today _____ Ⓜ Ⓣ Ⓦ Ⓣ Ⓕ Ⓢ Ⓢ

Muscle Group Focus _____ Weight _____ Date/Time _____

Stretch ○ Warm-Up _____

Strength Training

Exercise	Set	1	2	3	4	5	6	7
	Reps							
	Weight							
	Reps							
	Weight							
	Reps							
	Weight							
	Reps							
	Weight							
	Reps							
	Weight							
	Reps							
	Weight							
	Reps							
	Weight							
	Reps							
	Weight							

Cardio

Exercise	Calories	Distance	Time

Water intake _____

Cooldown _____

Feeling ☆☆☆☆☆

Notes

Goals for Today _____   Ⓜ Ⓣ Ⓦ Ⓣ Ⓕ Ⓢ Ⓢ

Muscle Group Focus _____   Weight _____   Date/Time _____

Stretch ○   Warm-Up _____

Strength Training

Exercise	Set	1	2	3	4	5	6	7
	Reps							
	Weight							
	Reps							
	Weight							
	Reps							
	Weight							
	Reps							
	Weight							
	Reps							
	Weight							
	Reps							
	Weight							
	Reps							
	Weight							
	Reps							
	Weight							

Cardio

Exercise	Calories	Distance	Time
_____			
_____			
_____			
_____			

Water intake _____

Cooldown _____

Feeling ☆☆☆☆☆

Notes

Body Measurement

Date/Period							
Weight							
Body Fat %							
Neck							
Shoulders							
Chest							
Bicep Right							
Bicep Left							
Forearm Right							
Forearm Left							
Wrist							
Waist							
Hips							
Thigh Right							
Thigh Left							
Calf Right							
Calf Left							

Goals

Description	Deadline

Thank you!

WE ARE GLAD THAT YOU PURCHASED OUR BOOK!
PLEASE LET US KNOW HOW WE CAN IMPROVE IT!
YOUR FEEDBACK IS ESSENTIAL TO US.

Contact us at:

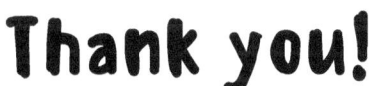 log'Sin@gmail.com

---

JUST TITLE THE EMAIL 'CREATIVE' AND WE WILL GIVE YOU SOME EXTRA SURPRISES!